So You're Dating a Psychopath
Now What?

By Michele Gilbert

Visit My Amazon Author Page

Dedicated to those who choose to stretch beyond their own limits and seek an abundant and fulfilling life.

Your thoughts are creative.

Michele Gilbert

Table of contents

Introduction

So You Found Someone... Odd...

Is it a Sociopath?

The Point of No Return

The Nature of the Beast

What To Do

Getting On With Your Life

Conclusion

Introduction

I want to thank you and congratulate you for downloading the book, *So You're Dating a Psychopath: Now What?*

This book contains proven steps and strategies on how to fully comprehend and understand the basic traits and issues of those suffering from psychopathy and how to deal with it.

There are thousands of people out there that are afflicted with psychopathy, as many as one in twenty five. So what happens if you think the person you're dating or are involved with is a psychopath? By picking up this book, you're on your way to identifying and handling the situation accordingly. It's a scary topic and we're here to help.

This book will help you distinguish the difference between psychopaths and sociopaths and why they're similar. You'll be given inside knowledge into how psychopaths tick and what they truly are. There will be a step by step guide on how to get out of a relationship if you're in one with a psychopath. It's all right here, waiting for you to discover.

So are you ready?

Then let's begin the journey...

So You Found Someone... Odd...

So here's an interesting situation. Life hasn't been so great. Work is fine and your finances are pretty good, but your love life isn't exactly the greatest thing ever. But there's something on the horizon. There's a guy or a girl that you can't help but feel is absolutely perfect. They're the missing piece. They're the best thing that you've ever found. But there's just something off. There's something that just doesn't seem right to you.

They seem odd.

Now, that's something that just doesn't seem right to you. It's something that really makes you question whether you're looking to sabotage this yourself or if you're really seeing a problem. The issue is that it's so ethereal; it's so nebulous that you're not sure what it is that is wrong with this person. You just look at all the peaces of your relationship and you think that maybe it's you. Maybe it's you who is ruining this.

But maybe it's not.

Sure, that's a valid point, a lot of people do sabotage the relationships they're in and taking the moment to look at your own approach to your relationships is an important step in figuring out whether you're the root of this strange feeling you're having. But let's say that you're a reasonable person and that's exactly what you do. You come to the conclusion that it's you and that there's a pretty great person in your life and you should be grateful for them. But, in the end, you're not the person who is sabotaging this. No one is sabotaging this, there's just something off.

Maybe it's because the whole thing is a lie.

That's right, an illusion that's being projected.

So here's the deal, you need to be certain before going beyond this point. You have tried everything, you have searched yourself and your mysterious partner, and this is the end. There's no going past this point. This is the Point of No Return. After this, you're going to see an ugly truth. Beyond this point, you're going to come to one of two conclusions. The first conclusion is that you're absolutely insane and paranoid. You're the person here who needs to get real and see that you've got a problem. But, the other conclusion that you're probably going to come to is unnerving and terrifying.

The person you're dating might be a psychopath.

That's the horrifying truth that you might come to. Psychopaths are out there and they are living in society, just like the rest of us, living like the normal people we think they are. The most recent studies say that there is somewhere around twelve million psychopaths out there among us. They get this from four percent. Four percent of the population, that's four out of a hundred. One in twenty five. The reality of that is going to sink in when you think about it for a moment.

Are you dating a psychopath? How can you tell?

Now, if you really think that you might be dating a psychopath, then go to the next chapter. Go to the next chapter and see if your suspicions are true. However, if you think that there's something else that might be wrong, that you're not dating a psychopath. Then be warned, this is the point of no return, because you're going to find out some hard truths about yourself in this book if it turns out that you're wrong. So here you go. Here's the rabbit hole. Here's the point of no return for you.

Is it a Sociopath?

Alright, if we go one step forward, let's take a moment to see if there's something you think you know or if you need to know. There's a difference between psychopaths and sociopaths. There's a huge difference and you need to know what you're dealing with, so let's clear some of the murky waters that might be messing with your read on the situation right now. So let's get down to brass tacks. What's a psychopath and what's a sociopath?

Well, without spoiling the rest of the book, let's just take some time to talk about what sociopaths are. Sociopaths are about as common as psychopaths are and that makes them just as scary. Like psychopaths, they're social butterflies and they're extremely good at reading people. Sociopaths are found all over in society but often do not concede to one group that they are most prevalent in. They cannot form emotional attachments with people and also lack the traditional value system that psychopaths also lack.

In the end, there's a reason why psychopaths and sociopaths are mistaken for each other. However, there is an extreme difference that makes psychopaths infinitely more terrifying.

Sociopaths have a skewed value system, which means that there is a preexisting value system, but that it is not normal like most people. With serious therapy and a conscious effort to change, sociopaths can be given a chance to change who they are. Psychopaths need invasive help and sometimes surgery to change who they are. This value system means that sociopaths can often be catered to or made to see what they are doing is wrong in often a bizarre or paradoxical way. If you can genuinely negotiate with the person you suspect of being a psychopath and barter with them on giving you up, then they're probably a sociopath.

Now here is the real difference that should be alarming to anyone dealing with a psychopath, only a very small number of murderers or serial killers are listed as sociopaths. In the end, sociopaths my think terrible things or how easy it would be to harm someone, but rarely do they perform. When dealing with a sociopath, the risk to yourself is very high, but it is still lower than if you're dealing with a psychopath.

Those are the two main differences between a psychopath and a sociopath. One, a sociopath has a value system, although it is seriously faulting or lacking in moral alignment. Second, a sociopath will only rarely move to harm you physically. So before we continue on, here are two things you know up front about psychopaths from what sociopaths' lack.

First, they do not have a value or moral system.

Second, they will harm you and do not filter violence.

This means that when we go forward and you're certain that the person you're dealing with is a psychopath, then you need to keep these things in mind for your own sake. Things are serious when you start diagnosing people as psychopaths, so be prepared for the consequences of what this means if you are truly involved with a psychopath.

Alright, let's keep moving.

The Point of No Return

Okay, so you're fairly certain that you're dating a psychopath. You're like ninety percent sure. You're so certain that you're reading a book about psychopaths to see what a psychopath truly looks like. You're that certain. Okay, fair enough. So here's what I'm going to call the point of no return. You're so certain that you're here and that's totally fine. You should feel completely okay with that.

So here's what we know about psychopathy.

It's Common:

Here's a few numbers for you. If you're a guy reading this book, thinking that your wife or girlfriend might be a psychopath, then there's a good chance that they're not. Studies indicate that one percent of women are actually psychopaths. However, if you think that the mysterious man in your life might be a psychopath, the numbers are in the favor of men. Three percent of men are considered to be psychopaths. Those numbers are fairly terrifying.

Psychopathy is a common condition among people and these are people who are out in the world, roaming around like you and eye. This isn't something that you should be afraid of. Pretty much all of these people have no idea that they're psychopaths themselves. It's just good to know that there are numbers out here about this. So, don't be afraid, just know: they're out there. It's common enough to be alarming, but don't be scared of it.

They Don't Know What They Are:

Most psychopaths are undiagnosed and have absolutely no idea what they are. That means that they're wandering around, completely clueless of what they are. There are plenty of ways for you to pick up on if the person you're dating is a psychopath, but we'll come to that later. What you need to know about this is that the person you're probably thinking is a psychopath, they probably have no clue. Now, if you find out that they do know they're a psychopath, then all bets are off. Get rid of them and run for the hills as fast as you can.

Now, if the person you're dating is incredible, is everything you're looking for, and is a wonderful person, they just sow off some strange and disturbing traits, then have mercy on them. Have some kindness and decency in your heart and try approaching them. Break it to them nicely. We'll go over this in a later chapter, but keep this in mind. Just because the person you're dating is a psychopath, that doesn't mean that they're going to chop you up and eat you for dinner.

It's Worked Out Pretty Well So Far:

Here's the problem with psychopaths and telling them that they have a problem. Before they've actually committed a crime, psychopathy has probably given them an edge in the world. Sure, it's a debilitating disorder and it makes them a danger to themselves, those they know, and society, but that doesn't mean that it hasn't given them an edge. A lot of great successes in society have been psychopaths and a lot of shrewd, cutthroat businessmen are psychopaths. People who have a vision of what they want and pursue it wholeheartedly without having any remorse about who gets burned or hurt along the way, they're probably psychopaths. Now, this gives them the advantage of being extremely efficient, ruthless, and successful. So, be aware of what you might be stripping from them when you bring up the fact that they might be psychopaths. It's going to be a hard sell.

It Is All a Lie:

Here's the hard truth. Now, you really want this person to be what you think they are: charming, warm, friendly, driven, and passionate; but the reality is that psychopaths usually are not this way. The truth is that the person you think that you've fallen in love with is probably nothing more than a portrait that they have painted custom for you. Psychopaths, whether they know what they are or not, know that society has standards and ideas that they want and they've identified them early on. They know that you're looking for something specific and like an article of clothing; they've put on everything you want and need. If you feel like the speed in which you discovered things about what they love and are interested in feels almost magical, that might be the case.

Lying and manipulation is the key indicator of a psychopath. They have no remorse, no fear, and their empathy is flipped on like a switch inside their brains. There is nothing real about the persona they've built for you and there is probably no knowing who they really are, because most psychopaths don't know themselves who they are. They know only their desires and their wants and that dictates exactly who they are. Outside of their wants, they probably do not know who they are. It is a hollow emptiness that they try to fill with accomplishments and successes, little victories that they've achieved.

You may just be another little victory that they're trying to tuck away and if that's the case, there may be no going back.

Why this is the Point of No Return:

Do not be a Harley Quinn and do not love your Joker without thought or without consequence. When it comes to psychopaths, they are destructive. They build worlds that are not real and when they tear them down, it is devastating and it is harmful. Psychopaths can act violently without fear or regret and there is a lot at stake in your life other than your physical personage that they can target. This means that you're going to need to be careful from this point on out if you're certain that you're dealing with a psychopath.

The reason why this is the point of no return is that everything I've just told you adds up. They don't know that they're a psychopath, they're not going to want to change, and everything that they know about themselves and you know about them is a lie. The most tempting thing you're going to want to do with this information is confront the person you're suspecting of being a psychopath, but I'm telling you not to.

I'm telling you to fade away. Don't be bold, don't be dramatic, and don't be hostile. Just tell them that you're not into this relationship anymore or that you're just going to need some time to explore you. Find a simple, understandable reason for needing to separate and make it amicable. Because, this is the point of no return. You're not going to be able to salvage this and love is not going to conquer this. In fact, things are probably going to get worse if you don't do as I suggest.

So that's why this is the point of no return. That's why all of these things add up to a really big problem and if you're sensing that's something's wrong and you've exhausted all the possibilities up to this point, then you might want to take a deep breath and see if you want to keep going. If you think that the key to all of this might be that there are a lot of lies in your home and life, then you're probably dealing with a psychopath. Seriously, dear reader, this is the harbinger of the end for you.

The Nature of the Beast

So what is a psychopath what do they look like and what should you be suspecting from the future? These are all fair questions and these are all people that we should want to be able to identify in our lives as we go around. So I've got a list here that will hopefully narrow some of the specific traits that you're looking for down. Have a look and see if the person you have in mind is racking up the check marks for you

A Lack of Fear:

This manifests itself in a whole bunch of ways. A lack of fear can mean that they're willing to take risks and gamble things that are often of high value that others will not risk. This doesn't mean that they're successful or that they have a penchant for victory, but rather that they stand out. This might bring them success in the business world for being "ballsy" or "having the guts to do what's necessary" but that's not really a good thing when it's applied to every aspect of their life and it is. A true psychopath will gamble anything because they are not afraid of the response that is registered or applied to them.

So this means that they're extremely high risk. This can be appealing at first, because it can show them as carefree and reckless even or it can mean that they're adrenaline driven. They might be into extreme sports or gambling, which gives them a bad boy/bad girl appeal. Again, just because you're into extreme sports or gambling, doesn't mean you're a psychopath. It's just a trait that they have. This is going to show up, again, in every aspect of their life. They're not going to be afraid of consequences that would make you or I stop and hesitate. No matter how big or small, a psychopath won't flinch.

There are examples of when they will show what look like signs of being afraid. Psychopaths are excellent manipulators and when you're watching, they're going to put on the show for you. If they know that you're on to them or that they need to act afraid in certain moments, they will. This is just a show and the moment you're out of sight, they'll switch it off.

All of this is caused by a part of the brain that studies are beginning to reveal as the source of this problem. It all stems from the amygdala, which is a part of the brain that regulates fear. When you stop and break down fear, it's just interpreting the consequences of loss. By judging something as valuable, the thought of losing it is comprehended by our mind as fear and that's all regulated by the amygdala. So by having an abnormal amygdala or having a tumor growing there as many do, this interferes with their lives in the manifestation of psychopathy. So without fear, they're willing to risk everything and give up everything.

Why Fear Matters:

Fear is a good thing. Fear is probably the one thing that helps regulate your life better than any other emotion that you have. Fear is what tells you your priorities, your values, and your concerns. Fear keeps you safe and alive. Though too much fear often hinders and cripples us, a life without fear is infinitely worse, because a life without fear means that you have no value and this is what is revealed about psychopaths.

They have no value.

There is nothing in their life that they're going to consider worth being afraid of losing. A psychopath is smoke and mirrors and when you get to the bottom of it, they lack value and respect for things. This fearlessness is a clear indicator that there is something wrong with them. Without this, they are often incapable of love, care, and will disregard the feelings of others to achieve whatever it is that they've set their mind to conquering.

The only thing that they do value is the illusion of value.

The Great Lie:

Now, here's where things start to get tricky, and they're extremely tricky with psychopaths. The one thing that psychopaths all have in common is the drive inside of them. Their lack of value and connection to things or entities around them creates a vacuum inside of them that they're desperate to fill. Whether it's through violence toward people or the acquisition of things they think will slake their thirst for more, Psychopaths are living under the illusion that there is something out there that will make them happy.

Most commonly among psychopaths, this mirage they're chasing is professional success. Psychopaths will fixate upon something that they think they need. It might be you, that promotion, a new beach house, or a myriad of other things that they have made their objective. They will pursue it to achieve their goal by any means necessary and the moment that goal is achieved, they move on to something else. Unsatisfied and disappointed by their previous objective, a psychopath will often show his hand at the moment where you're no longer what he/she wants anymore.

Anger:

Now, if a psychopath has accomplished his/her goal in acquiring you as a boyfriend or girlfriend, then you're going to start noticing some things. The first and foremost is anger. It starts out as frustration and irritability, but it will quickly develop into more if you're not careful. Picking a fight with a psychopath is the worst thing you could do, because they're going to be all in.

Remember, no fear or value. If you're noticing that obstacles in this person-you're-suspecting's way are provoking outrage or just outbursts, these are definite psychopathic attributes. Of course, make sure that the situation doesn't warrant it. If you're partner explodes because they got undercut in a promotion or just lost a huge client, anger is an inappropriate, but understandable response to this. We're talking about someone forgetting to send a memo or them getting a stain on their shirt at lunch before a meeting. If this provokes a hostile, angry response, then there's a problem.

Of course, psychopaths have a whole slew of ticks and this is just one of them, one that you're most likely to take note of at first. This second sign is far more insidious and destructive.

The Lies:

Psychopaths know that there is something off about them, but they're not overly concerned about it. What they're afraid of is being seen as different or someone recognizing that there is something wrong about them. So in order to hide this, they begin constructing an intricate web of lies that goes very deep.

In order to define yourself as a human being, you need to know what it is that you stand for and value in life. Mediation, contemplation, and spiritual pursuits often lead us to the core of our lives and touch what it means to be truly you. However, without value or something that you stand upon, you cannot truly know who you are or what it is that means the most to you. Without that, you're left hollow and wanting. So a psychopath is truly left hollow and needs to compensate. So they begin to build a personality to replace the one that they do not have. This takes on the form of lies and half-truths.

Like I told you earlier to have mercy and be understanding about the person who might be a psychopath in your life, but be willing to see them for what they are, this is why. Everything you know about them, or you think you know about them is a lie. Your relationship's foundation is a lie. Their actions are motivated by a desire to get you—to acquire you, not by love. This web of lies that they've spun goes deep into their core being and you cannot find true intimacy with them because there is nothing there. They do not have something for you to connect with. You're grasping at phantom hands.

So if they're all lies, smoke and mirrors, then how can you tell? How can you tell that they're a psychopath? If they're that good at lying, is there really a way for you to ever truly know? Yes and here's how.

The Charm and Seduction:

Psychopaths know that they need to put on a face for society and that means that they're students of behavior. They have been watching and reading people since they first realized that they don't quite fit in. This means that they have a hand crafted and sculpted personality without any of the flaws that you or I have. This means that they're extremely charming and seductive when you're talking to them. They're the freaking Borg of society. With every failure, they regroup and try again with another victim. They tailor their responses and reactions to everything until it's a formula that they can apply to anyone that they meet.

If the person you suspect of being a psychopath is charming and seductive to you, knew all the right moves and knew exactly what to say, that's a really bad sign. There isn't a single psychopath out there that can't make you like them, or worse, fall in love with you.

This is manipulation at its finest and it will run deeper and deeper into your life if you let it and soon, they'll start jerking on the cords they've hooked into you and see if they can make you dance.

They Want to Test the Waters:

So they're so charming and so wonderful that they've hooked you in and one thing that all psychopaths do is want to know that they're succeeding. They don't want unreadable data. They need to know whether they're wasting their time or not and that's only visible if they can register some kind of a response out of you. The response that they love most and they like to try the best is pity.

To see if you are actually buying into the lies that they're selling you or to see if you're caught, they need to manipulate you. They need to see if they can trigger some kind of response and pity makes them feel good at the same time, furthering their goals. It's a threefold maneuver on their part. They're testing the strength they have over you at this point, establish an emotional victory on their part, and make your emotional investment deepen with them. Essentially, they're pulling you deeper down the rabbit hole that they've built for you.

These little pity movements are going to happen whenever you might fight with them, might discover a lie, or might suspect something is amiss. They'll reestablish their dominance and their security with you by accidentally hurting themselves, being wronged some way in society, or do something perceived as heroic that causes them agony or suffering. If you're finding yourself feeling bad or pitying this person, then you're probably being manipulated and tested by a psychopath.

This will clash with the next trait I'm going to reveal to you that often gives them the stance of being a martyr in your or their eyes. They are often 'wronged' by those around you. Often justice or consequences of their actions will be spun as wrongs committed upon them. All of this is being used to see how you will react and how invested you are in their lie.

Of course, this can happen on multiple levels within their minds. They can be subconsciously doing this to you or they may be openly and knowingly manipulating you. It's usually somewhere between knowing and it just being what they do at this point in their life. Just be aware of it.

King of the World:

Here's a sad and scary fact all rolled up into one: psychopaths are often highly intelligent. This usually comes in the form of untapped potential or underutilized potential. They're smart and they know it. They might just be smart in a narrow field, or what they're specifically interested in, or everything, it really depends upon the person. The point is that they're smart and this breeds an unavoidable trait within someone who is both highly intelligent and someone who lacks a moral standing.

It's a god complex.

Depending upon the severity of the complex that they have, they will often see themselves as superior to everyone, including you. They will take any chance they can to demonstrate their intelligence to you with subtle stabs toward how you're not. Again, this is going to really hit home when they're playing the pity card. They will come across as victims, martyrs and various other forms of the unjustly wronged of society.

There is going to be something disappointing and alarming by how smug and superior they're going to see themselves. They're charismatic, fearless, and they're smart. This gives them the flare for the dramatic and that's going to really highlight their superiority. They're the best, they're the most dangerous and they're going to make sure that you know it.

Fallen Gods:

Because this is completely unrealistic, because last time I checked, there isn't a king of the world, they have unrealistic goals. So if you're looking for signs that you're dating a psychopath, are they always failing? Because they set themselves on the pedestal and think that they are gods, psychopaths are always going to find themselves failing. They can't shoot for the moon, because they might be smart, they might be charming, and they might be great at lying, but they're not everything they see themselves as. This is a recipe for disaster and it shows.

They fail constantly because their goals are not realistic and their goals are not going to work for them. In truth, there's nothing that's going to work out for them when they work for things they can't succeed at. See how this feeds into their pity/martyrdom desires? They shoot for these lofty, idealistic goals and then they fail horribly then spin that into seeing if you're going to feel sorry for them. Of course, they're also going to get angry about how they fail or how everything gets in their way. It's horrible. It's manipulative and it feeds a beast that will never be satisfied and you're just a gear in the machine.

They see themselves as fallen gods and they're looking to you to validate them and it's all a lie. You're being turned into a victim and you don't even know it yet.

What To Do

So if this list of everything terrible and dark that's all about psychopath is shooting of red lights like you're in some shady part of Amsterdam, then you're definitely wondering right about now what it is you're supposed to do about all of this. Either you're discarding this book or you're freaking out. Take a moment, if you're freaking out and let this just sink in. It's okay to be terrified and it's totally okay to feel a little overwhelmed by all of this. But in the end, you're going to have to make some tough decisions.

First of all, you're going to need to tell someone you trust about what you think you've discovered. No matter what happens to you from this moment on, you're going to need a rock to help you. If you at any point feel in danger or scared by what's happening to you, then you need someone who can get you out of there no matter the time or situation. You need to have that rock, that stability, and that dependability.

Second, you need to start making your exit plan. Let me tell you something right now and get it through your head without any doubt in your mind:

You cannot fix this!

You are not qualified because you need to understand that. There is no fixing this, there is no salvaging this, and there is nothing in the cards that you can play to save this. This is a sinking ship and it's going down, they don't know it and you don't know it. This ship is going down and no matter what you're hoping to do; it's not going to work out for you. If you confront them, they will get violent or they will lie to you. They are going to manipulate you and deceive you into believing that they'll change, but they'll lie to you all along the way. There is no fixing this and you do not have the resources to even try for it.

The third thing you need to know is that psychopaths are violent by their angry nature. There is a vast difference between sociopaths and psychopaths. We're dealing with a psychopath here and when their backs are against the wall, the main difference between psychopaths and sociopaths is that they will hurt you. They will harm you and they will not think anything about it. They will harm you and you need to be aware of that. You need to be prepared for that possibility, so avoid it entirely. Do not confront them. Do not tell them that they are psychopaths and do not confront them about this. That's not a fight that you want to get into this.

Fourthly, be prepared to do whatever is necessary. Psychopaths are liars, as we've established. They're more than willing to do whatever is necessary to deceive those who are invested in them. They will tell you that they're getting better, but unless you put a GPS tracking device on them, there's no way to know whether or not they're telling the truth. Assume the worst, because they're a psychopath. So when everything goes south and you know that there's no coming back from it, then you need to be willing to do whatever is necessary to get out of there.

When you're away from them, there's really no knowing what they're going to do. They might just let you go. Their goals might have moved on to someone or something different. When it comes to dealing with psychopaths, you're going to need to be ready to call the police, to call friends for help, to move if you have to, or do whatever is necessary to get on with your life. That's this final, fourth point for you. Be prepared to do whatever you're going to need to do to get away from this psychopath.

Getting On With Your Life

You have had the worst luck of anyone who has ever walked this earth and that's the sad fact that you've been entrapped in the web of lies spun by a psychopath. It sucks, I know. But that doesn't mean that you're the only person out there who has suffered from this and there are people out there that can help you. You are not alone.

Remember that there's a whole bunch of people out there who can help you and there's a lot resources at your disposal for getting to the point in your life where you feel safe to move on. I will tell you this right now, do not remain sentimental or tied to this person in any way. Think of them as poison infecting your life right now. You need to get it out as quickly as possible and that can only happen if you're willing to do whatever is necessary.

If you find yourself forgotten by your psychopath, then you're extremely lucky. You're able to move on rather easily. It's nice to be in that kind of a position because you'll be rather easy to get away from them.

However, if you're dealing with someone who is not very happy with losing you, then you're kind of stuck with a tag along monster for a while. Here's what you need to do.

If they show up, call the police. Don't mess around with this one. Call the police at any sign of your personal psychopath. The police will show up and help you at any point. It would be smart to start the application for a restraining order if you feel worried about yourself and your safety. Psychopaths will not just focus on you, they will utilize the fact that you do care about people. They will harm or work to harm anyone or anything that you value. They're willing to play dirty and they're willing to harm anything you love. So get a restraining order if you feel in danger. Don't wait for something terrible to happen. Be proactive about it. Protect the things you love.

If they're not turning violent, but you just can't shake them. Try manipulating them away from you. Unfortunately for psychopaths who are so willing to lie and manipulate those they know, they're also super easy to manipulate. Cater to the things that they often focus on. By this point, you should know that they're interested in achieving their goals, so try to turn them on to their other goals and desires. Get them to focus on things other than you. Try as hard as you can to get them interested in something else.

Finally, just be willing to protect yourself and get away from them. Psychopaths are not humorous or a joke. If you truly think that you're dealing with a psychopath, then you need to be willing to do what is necessary to get your life back in order. It's not going to be fun or easy, but I promise you that you'll be able to find a point where you can escape the horrors and the troubles of living and dealing with a psychopath. Eventually, you're going to be able to find a point in your life where you can move on. It'll be hard work, it'll be scare, and it will be absolutely worth it.

Take a deep breath and do what you need to do.

Conclusion

I hope this book was able to help you to understand a little more about Psychopaths.

The next step is to do whatever it is to see if you're dating a psychopath and now you know how to get away!

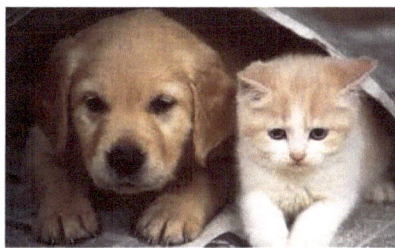

Before you go, I'd like to say thank you for purchasing my book.

I know you could have picked so many other books to read on life with a psychopath. But you took a chance on me.

So A Big thanks for downloading this book and reading it all the way to completion.

Now I would like to ask a _small_ favor.

Could you please take a minute or two to leave a review for this book on Amazon?

Click here

The feedback will help me continue to publish more kindle books that will help people to get better results in their lives.

And if you found it helpful in anyway then please let me know :-)

Thank you and good luck!

To your success,

Michele

Preview of My New Book

The Verbal And Emotional Abuser: Recognizing The Verbal Abusive Relationship And How To Defend Yourself

CHAPTER 1
Understanding an Abuser

Humans are complicated and complex beings. From the very moment of our birth, we interact with countless other people. How we turn out as unique individuals is a result of numerous unseen factors like genetics and subtle environmental cues. We also are shaped by the social environments in which we grow and mature. Which one of these factors affects our development more is a matter of contention among psychologists and scientists alike. The nature v. nurture argument shows no sign of letting up anytime soon. These essential realities of our identity and how we become who we are cannot be denied.

However, sometimes an individual, for a myriad of reasons, can evolve into an abusive person. It is a well-established fact that many abusive individuals are products of abuse themselves. David M. Allen, M.D. says "While it is important to realize that not all abusers were abused as children, and that many if not most people who are abused do not go on to become abusers themselves, child abuse is most likely the single largest factor - biological, psychological, or sociological - for later adult abusive behavior." In this respect, many abusers are victims of abuse and cannot be judged without keeping that simple fact in mind.

If someone close to you is verbally abusive, then there is a strong likelihood that at some point during their life they experienced physical, verbal, emotional, or sexual abuse. If you are in a position to do so, it might be beneficial to discover more about why the abuser close to you behaves in the manner in which they do. They may be reluctant to open up to you about these experiences, as the experiences have caused them a lot of trauma and pain. If they are open to the possibility, then suggest seeing a therapist. If they are willing to seek professional help, then be supportive in their pursuit to find healing. But if your attempts to understand the abuser close to you are fruitless, and they are unwilling to seek professional help, then the only thing left to understand is how abusers become the abusive individuals they are.

Although abuse during childhood is a common trait of abusive individuals, as mentioned before, it is not present on every case of an abusive individual. However, just because an abuser wasn't abused physically doesn't mean there wasn't any dysfunction in their upbringing. Familial dysfunction can manifest in many various forms. For example, emotional abuse can be very subtle and hard to spot. Furthermore, subtle emotional abuse can sometimes be repressed or difficult to remember. Emotional abuse is not always as obvious as yelling, insulting, or threatening speech. Emotional abuse can take the form of passive-aggressive speech, unhealthy comparisons ("You're not as pretty as your sister" or "If only you were as smart as your brother"), or even emotional neglect.

Abusive manifestations like these, especially passive aggressive speech and emotional neglect, can take their toll on a young child. But they may not have a conscious bearing on their mind. Or, in other words, these abusive behaviors may have been interpreted by the abused as normal behavior. In fact, they may blame themselves for this behavior. This self-blame is true for the physically abused, as well. It is important to understand abuse as a cycle. Abuse is a cycle that often repeats itself. It may change forms or focus, however. For example, an abused child may continue the cycle of abuse during adulthood, but not by abusing another, but by abusing themselves in the form of alcohol or drug abuse and self-harm. Knowing all this, it is possible that even the abuser in your life is willing to talk to you about the abusive experiences in their past, they may not know the full extent of the abuse.

If this is the case, then the best strategy is to try to understand as much as possible about the nature of their upbringing. How was their relationship with their parents? Often, abusive individuals were influenced negatively by the presence of a narcissistic individual. Due to the controlling and emotionally manipulative qualities of a narcissist, children raised by narcissists are sometimes subjected to emotional or physical abuse. However, it is important to note that not every narcissist is physically, or even emotionally, abusive. There are a multitude of personality disorders that a parent or close loved-one might have that could contribute to a child's abusive behavior later in life.

Unfortunately, you don't have to be a narcissist or have a personality disorder to cause damage in a child's life- the kind of damage that goes on to influence their actions as abusers. Neglecting a child emotionally, while not necessarily abusive, can be very detrimental to a child and can contribute to later abusive behavior. So, what is neglect? Well, neglect can be as simple as not acknowledging the child's importance. For the neglectful parent, they can simply not put a priority on the time they spend, if it exists at all, with their children. People who spend more time in the office than with their children can put their children at risk for emotional immaturity. This immaturity can preclude them towards being abuse. However, don't forget that some parents are intentionally neglectful and make it a point to disregard their children's emotional needs. In these cases especially, a child's emotional development can shed light on why they have become abusers themselves.

Without a doubt, an abusers childhood and upbringing have a lot to do with why they behave in an abusive manner. However, childhood abuse is not the only source for an abusive individual's behavior. Drug and alcohol abuse are significant factors, as well. There are also many factors like genetics, hormonal imbalances, or even nutritional deficiencies that can increase aggressive behavior. However, every individual is different. As mentioned elsewhere, each of these common traits of an abusive individual could be present in someone who has never engaged in abusive behavior. All in all, what distinguishes an abuser is their abusive behavior that is directed towards themselves or others.

CHAPTER 2
The Consequences of Abuse

Understanding why someone might behave in an abusive manner is the first step towards liberating yourself from these individuals. If your partner is the abusive individual, then there is an added level of urgency to the matter. However, in situations such as these, it is not merely enough to understand why or how they became abusers. It is equally, if not more important, to understand what happens to ourselves as a recipient of abuse at the hands of our partner or someone close to you.

Click Here To Check Out The Rest Of

The Verbal And Emotional Abuser: Recognizing The Verbal Abusive Relationship And How To Defend Yourself

P.S. You'll find many more books like this and others under my name Michele Gilbert.

Don't miss them... here is a short list.

Stop Playing Mind Games: How To Free Yourself Of Controlling And Manipulating Relationships

Instant Charisma: A Quick And Easy Guide To Talk, Impress, And Make Anyone Like You

Chakras: Understanding The 7 Main Chakras For Beginners: The Ultimate Guide To Chakra Mindfulness, Balance and Healing

Practicing Mindfulness: Living in the moment through Meditation: Everyday Habits and Rituals to help you achieve inner peace

Sleep Tight: Overcome Insomnia and Sleep Disorders for a better more restful sleep!

Stop Back Pain Now!: Back Pain Remedies and Treatments so you can live a pain free life!

The Arthritis Pain Cure: How to find Arthritis Pain Relief and live a happy pain free life!

The Headache Pain Cure: How to find Headache Pain Relief and live a happy Pain Free Life!

Stop Panic Attacks and Anxiety Disorders without Drugs Now!: Overcome Panic, Stress and Anxiety and live a happy pain free life!

The Breakup Recovery Guide: Advice for Surviving Heartbreak, Letting Go and Thriving in an exciting new life!

The Friendship Guide to Finding Friends Forever: How to Find, Make and Keep Quality Friendships After your Breakup

The Credit Fix: Leave behind credit card debt and poor credit scores and get your life back!

How To Stop Being Jealous And Insecure: Overcome Insecurity And Relationship Jealousy

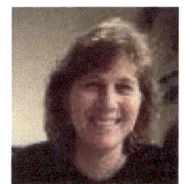

Michele Gilbert was born and raised in Brooklyn, New York. Drawn to literature and writing at a young age, she enrolled at Brooklyn College and majored in English. After graduation Michele did not begin writing immediately, instead she embarked on a career in the finance industry and spent the next thirty years on Wall Street.

Serendipity struck when she least expected it. After ending a long-term relationship, Michele found herself lost and unsure what the future held. She began to read books on grief and loss, looking for answers. Those led her to delve deeper into the Law of Attraction and its power. What resulted was remarkable. Not only had she begun to heal, she had also rekindled her former love of writing and discovered her life's purpose.

The years have taken her through many twists and turns, but she learned valuable lessons along the way. Today she publishes books-mostly self-help and metaphysical in nature-and feels compelled to share her knowledge with those facing similar experiences. Her greatest hope is to inspire others and show them ways to overcome adversity and gracefully accept life's inevitable low points.

Going forward, she plans to incorporate more teachings of self-help, finance and meditation. Regular meditation is very beneficial to her progress as she forges a new life. Morning rituals and positive incantations are other practices Michele embraces; they are very restorative in daily life. As an avid hiker, Michele and fellow club members often hike the picturesque Jersey Pine Barrens. She is a history buff, voracious reader, baseball fanatic and a foodie. She also proudly supports Trout Unlimited-a national non-profit organization dedicated to conserving, protecting and restoring North America's Coldwater fisheries and their watersheds.

Michele currently resides forty minutes from Atlantic City and the Jersey Shore. She makes her home with a Blue Russian rescue cat named Jersey, though she isn't exactly sure who rescued who.

Michele really enjoys publishing books that can make a difference in people's lives. If you have any suggestions or would like to have a specific topic covered in a future book, please send an email to michelegilbertbooks@gmail.com and we will get back to you.

Thanks for reading!